# HYPERTHYROIDISM SMOOTHIES BOOK

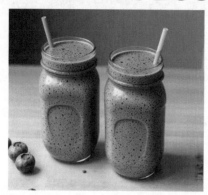

## 60 Delicious Smoothie Recipes To Manage Your Health Naturally

KELLY . D. LYONS

# THE COPYRIGHT PAGE

**Copyright © 2024 Kelly D. Lyons All rights reserved.**

2024.Kelly D. Lyons Reservation of rights. Except for brief quotations used in critical reviews and certain other noncommercial uses allowed by copyright law, no part of this publication may be duplicated, distributed, or transmitted in any way without the publisher's prior written consent. This prohibition includes photocopying, recording, and other electronic or mechanical methods

# TABLE OF CONTENT

# INTRODUCTION

## Understanding Hyperthyroidism

Hyperthyroidism is a medical condition that arises when the thyroid gland becomes overactive, producing excessive amounts of thyroid hormones. To truly grasp the significance of hyperthyroidism, it's essential to understand the pivotal role the thyroid gland plays in our bodies.

### *The Thyroid Gland: A Vital Regulator*

Imagine your thyroid gland as a small, butterfly-shaped organ situated in the front of your neck. Despite its unassuming size, the thyroid is a powerhouse, wielding immense control over various bodily functions. It serves as the body's metabolic thermostat, regulating how efficiently your cells convert nutrients into energy. This gland secretes two primary hormones, thyroxine (T4) and triiodothyronine (T3), which orchestrate a symphony of processes that influence your overall health.

## The Thyroid's Symphony

These thyroid hormones control your heart rate, breathing rate, body temperature, and the pace at which food is converted into energy. They also affect your mood, weight, and even the condition of your skin and hair. In essence, the thyroid is a master conductor, orchestrating the rhythm of life itself.

## The Causes of Hyperthyroidism

Hyperthyroidism can arise from various causes, with Graves' disease being the most common culprit. This autoimmune disorder occurs when the body's immune system mistakenly attacks the thyroid gland, prompting it to produce excessive hormones. Other causes include toxic multinodular goiter, thyroiditis, and certain medications or dietary supplements. It's essential to pinpoint the root cause to tailor the treatment effectively.

## The Symptoms

Living with hyperthyroidism can be challenging due to its wide array of symptoms. Imagine experiencing relentless fatigue despite a racing heart, anxiety that seems to have no cause, and unexplained weight loss despite an increased appetite. Additionally, you may find yourself sweating excessively, experiencing tremors, and battling muscle weakness. These symptoms can be disruptive and even alarming, underscoring the importance of early detection and management.

## *Sarah's Unexpected Journey*

Sarah's story serves as a poignant example of how hyperthyroidism can impact an individual's life. A vivacious and energetic woman in her early thirties, Sarah was known for her boundless enthusiasm and zest for life. Her friends marveled at her ability to tackle multiple projects, maintain an active social life, and excel in her career. Sarah was the embodiment of vitality, or so it seemed.

One summer, Sarah began to notice subtle changes in her body. Her heart rate seemed to quicken for no apparent reason, leaving her feeling jittery and anxious. She shrugged it off as stress initially, attributing her newfound restlessness to her demanding job. But as the weeks passed, the symptoms escalated. She experienced unexplained weight loss despite her love for hearty meals and began sweating profusely, even in air-conditioned rooms.

Concerned, Sarah sought medical advice. After a battery of tests, the diagnosis was clear – hyperthyroidism. The news was perplexing and unsettling for Sarah, who had always prided herself on her health-conscious lifestyle.

Sarah's journey towards understanding hyperthyroidism began with education. She delved into research, learning about the thyroid's vital role in regulating metabolism and overall health. As she delved deeper into the condition, she realized that the thyroid was intricately tied to nutrition.

## *The Power of Nutrition*

Nutrition is a cornerstone in the management of hyperthyroidism, and Sarah understood its importance. The right diet could help alleviate symptoms and support her journey toward recovery.

### *The Role of Nutrition in Hyperthyroidism*

Sarah discovered that certain nutrients played a pivotal role in thyroid health. Key among them were iodine and selenium, essential minerals that supported thyroid function. She also learned that cruciferous vegetables, such as broccoli and cauliflower, could potentially exacerbate her condition and decided to adjust her diet accordingly.

### Sarah Customizing Her Diet

Armed with knowledge, Sarah embarked on a mission to create a diet tailored to her condition. She incorporated iodine-rich foods like seafood, dairy, and eggs, and ensured her selenium intake was adequate. She also became adept at crafting smoothies with thyroid-supporting ingredients such as spinach, kale, and Brazil nuts, which she found not only delicious but also nourishing.

## Sarah's Transformation

Over time, Sarah's dedication to her diet paid off. Her energy levels stabilized, and her heart rate returned to a healthy rhythm. Her weight began to normalize, and she found a sense of balance she hadn't experienced in months.

Sarah's journey underscores the importance of understanding hyperthyroidism and the power of nutrition in managing this condition. By embracing knowledge and customizing her diet, she took control of her health and regained her vitality. Sarah's story serves as an inspiration to those facing hyperthyroidism, illustrating that with the right information and a tailored approach, one can overcome the challenges of this condition and enjoy a fulfilling life.

# ABOUT THE BOOK

**Do you suffer from hypothyroidism?**
**A condition that affects your thyroid gland and slows down your metabolism?**
**Do you want to boost your energy, lose weight, and improve your health with delicious and nutritious smoothies?**

*If you answered yes, then this book is for you*

*HYPERTHYROIDISM SMOOTHIES BOOK* is a comprehensive guide that will teach you how to make smoothies that nourish your thyroid and support your wellness. You will learn about the causes and symptoms of hyperthyroidism, the best ingredients to use in your smoothies, and the benefits of each one. You will also discover over 50 mouthwatering smoothie recipes that are easy to prepare and taste amazing. Each recipe has its photo, so you can see what your smoothie will look like before you make it.

*In this book, you will also find:*

- My personal story of how I overcame hyperthyroidism with smoothies
- Tips and guidelines for making smoothies that suit your preferences and needs

- Additional resources and references to help you learn more about hyperthyroidism and smoothies
- Testimonials and reviews from my readers and customers who have tried my smoothies and loved them

*HYPERTHYROIDISM SMOOTHIES BOOK* is more than just a cookbook. It is a lifestyle change that will help you feel better, look better, and live better. Whether you have hypothyroidism or not, you will enjoy these smoothies and reap their benefits.

But wait, there's more! If you order your copy of *HYPERTHYROIDISM SMOOTHIES BOOK* today, you will also get access to my other book, *HYPERTHYROIDISM SOLUTION COOKBOOK,* where you will find 80 more delicious recipes to manage your symptoms and transform your health.

Don't wait any longer. Order your copy of *HYPERTHYROIDISM SMOOTHIES BOOK* today and start blending your way to a healthier and happier you.

# Chapter :1

## What is Hyperthyroidism?

Hyperthyroidism is a medical condition characterized by the overproduction of thyroid hormones by the thyroid gland. The thyroid gland is a small, butterfly-shaped organ located in the front of your neck and plays a crucial role in regulating various bodily functions. Thyroid hormones, primarily thyroxine (T4) and triiodothyronine (T3), influence metabolism, energy production, heart rate, and many other essential processes.

## Causes of Hyperthyroidism:

**Several factors can contribute to the development of hyperthyroidism, including:**

*a) Graves' Disease:* The most common cause of hyperthyroidism is Graves' disease, an autoimmune disorder in which the body's immune system mistakenly attacks the thyroid gland, leading to excess hormone production.

*b) Toxic Multinodular Goiter:* This condition occurs when the thyroid gland develops multiple nodules, some of which produce thyroid hormones uncontrollably.

*c) Thyroiditis:* Inflammation of the thyroid gland can temporarily release stored hormones into the bloodstream, causing hyperthyroidism. This inflammation can result from infections or autoimmune disorders.

## *Symptoms of Hyperthyroidism:*

Hyperthyroidism can cause a wide range of symptoms, which may vary in severity among individuals. Common signs and *symptoms include:*

*Weight loss:* Despite increased appetite, individuals with hyperthyroidism often lose weight.
*Rapid heartbeat (tachycardia):*
An accelerated heart rate can lead to palpitations and irregular heart rhythms.
*Nervousness and anxiety:* Excessive thyroid hormones can make individuals feel jittery, anxious, or irritable.
*Sweating:* Increased perspiration and intolerance to heat are common.
*Fatigue:* Paradoxically, some people experience fatigue and weakness alongside hyperactivity.

*Tremors:* Fine tremors in the hands and fingers may occur.

*Muscle weakness:* Muscle weakness, particularly in the thighs and shoulders, can develop.

*Thinning hair and skin changes:* Hair may become brittle, and the skin may become thin and prone to bruising.

*Bulging eyes:* In Graves' disease, a condition called exophthalmos can cause the eyes to protrude.

*Menstrual irregularities:* Women with hyperthyroidism may experience changes in their menstrual cycles.

*Frequent bowel movements:* Diarrhea may result from increased gastrointestinal motility.

## How Hyperthyroidism Affects Your Health:

Hyperthyroidism, if left untreated, can have serious health consequences. It can lead to:

*Heart problems:* High levels of thyroid hormones can strain the heart and increase the risk of heart palpitations, high blood pressure, and arrhythmias.

*Osteoporosis:* Excessive thyroid hormone levels can cause bone loss, leading to osteoporosis and an increased risk of fractures.

*Eye problems:* In Graves' disease, eye problems such as double vision, eye pain, and vision changes can occur.

*Thyroid storm:* A rare but life-threatening complication of severe hyperthyroidism, characterized by high fever, rapid heartbeat, and confusion.

### Treatment Options for Hyperthyroidism:

Effective treatment for hyperthyroidism aims to normalize thyroid hormone levels and alleviate symptoms. Treatment options include:

*a) Medications:* Anti-thyroid medications like methimazole and propylthiouracil can reduce hormone production and are often used as a first-line treatment.

*b) Radioactive iodine therapy:* This treatment involves ingesting radioactive iodine, which selectively destroys overactive thyroid tissue.

*c) Surgery:* In some cases, surgical removal of part or all of the thyroid gland may be necessary, especially when other treatments are not suitable or fail.

*d)* *Beta-blockers:* These medications help manage symptoms like rapid heartbeat and anxiety.

*e)* *Monitoring:* Regular monitoring of thyroid function is essential to adjust treatment as needed and prevent complications.

## *Why Smoothies Are a Great Way to Nourish Your Thyroid and Boost Your Metabolism:*

Smoothies can be a beneficial addition to the diet of individuals with hyperthyroidism for several reasons:

*Nutrient Density:* Hyperthyroidism can lead to increased nutrient requirements, as the body is operating at a higher metabolic rate. Smoothies allow you to pack a variety of nutrient-dense ingredients into a single meal, ensuring you get essential vitamins, minerals, and antioxidants.

*Hydration:* Proper hydration is crucial for overall health and can help alleviate some of the symptoms of hyperthyroidism, such as sweating and diarrhea. Smoothies often contain hydrating ingredients like fruits and vegetables.

*Digestibility:* Digestive issues can accompany hyperthyroidism. Smoothies are easy to digest, making them suitable for individuals with sensitive stomachs or gastrointestinal symptoms.

*Balanced Nutrition:* Smoothies can be customized to provide a balanced mix of macronutrients, including protein, carbohydrates, and healthy fats, which are essential for overall health and energy balance.

*Fiber Content:* Adding fiber-rich ingredients like spinach, kale, or flaxseeds to your smoothie can support digestive health and help manage diarrhea, a common symptom of hyperthyroidism.

*Metabolism Boost:* Some ingredients used in smoothies, such as ginger, can help boost metabolism naturally, which may benefit those with an overactive thyroid.

*Hormone Regulation:* Certain ingredients, like Brazil nuts (rich in selenium), can support thyroid hormone regulation and balance.

## My Story of Overcoming Hyperthyroidism with Smoothies:

### Reclaiming My Health: How Smoothies Helped Me Overcome Hyperthyroidism "

For years, I struggled with the debilitating effects of hyperthyroidism. The constant fatigue, rapid heartbeat, and uncontrollable weight loss made me feel like a prisoner in my own body. Traditional treatments helped to some extent, but I yearned for a natural and empowering solution. That's when I discovered the incredible healing power of smoothies.

### How the Journey Begins:

My journey to overcoming hyperthyroidism with smoothies started with research. I delved into the science behind thyroid health and learned about the importance of nutrition in managing the condition. Armed with knowledge, I began experimenting with different ingredients and recipes.

### The Smoothie Transformation:

I soon realized that smoothies could be a game-changer. I started incorporating thyroid-supporting ingredients like spinach, kale, Brazil nuts and blueberries into my daily routine. These superfoods provided my body with the nutrients it desperately needed to regain balance.

As I continued with my smoothie regimen, I noticed a significant improvement in my symptoms. The excess weight loss stopped, my energy levels increased, and my anxiety began to subside. The hydrating properties of the smoothies helped counteract the constant sweating, and the fiber-rich ingredients eased my gastrointestinal discomfort.

What I loved most about my smoothie journey was the sense of empowerment it gave me. Instead of relying solely on medications, I took an active role in my health. I felt a deep connection to the healing power of nature and the nourishment it provided. Smoothies became not just a meal but a ritual of self-care.

Word spread about my progress, and friends and family began asking for my smoothie recipes. I shared my knowledge and recipes, witnessing their transformations as they embraced this holistic approach to managing hyperthyroidism.

Today, I stand as a testament to the healing potential of smoothies for thyroid health. Hyperthyroidism no longer controls my life, and I owe much of my recovery to the simple act of blending nutrient-rich ingredients into delicious and healing concoctions. I hope that my story inspires others to explore the benefits of smoothies in their journey toward better thyroid health.

## Tips and Guidelines for Making Delicious and Healthy Smoothies:

Creating delicious and healthy smoothies is easy when you follow these tips and guidelines:

### Choose Nutrient-Rich Ingredients:

Include a variety of fruits and vegetables like spinach, kale, berries, bananas, and avocados for vitamins, minerals, and antioxidants.

Incorporate sources of protein, such as Greek yogurt, tofu, or protein powder, to support muscle health.

Add healthy fats like almond butter, chia seeds, or flaxseeds for satiety and to support hormone balance.

### Hydration and Liquid Base:

Use liquids like water, coconut water, almond milk, or Greek yogurt as your base for proper hydration. Adjust the liquid quantity to achieve your preferred smoothie consistency.

## Balanced Macronutrients:

Aim for a balance of carbohydrates, protein, and fats in your smoothies to provide sustained energy. Customize your ratios based on your dietary preferences and nutritional needs.

## Sweeteners:

Use natural sweeteners like honey, maple syrup, or dates sparingly, as many fruits already provide natural sweetness.
Be mindful of added sugars in store-bought ingredients like flavored yogurt or fruit juices.

## Thyroid-Supporting Ingredients:

Incorporate thyroid-supporting foods like Brazil nuts (for selenium), seaweed (for iodine), and ginger (for metabolism support) into your smoothies.

## Fiber-Rich Additions:

Include fiber-rich ingredients like chia seeds, flaxseeds, or oats to aid digestion and promote satiety.

## Blending Technique:

Invest in a high-quality blender to ensure a smooth and creamy texture.
Start blending on low speed and gradually increase to avoid overwhelming the blender.

## Experiment and Customize:

Don't be afraid to experiment with different combinations of ingredients to find what you enjoy most.
Customize your smoothies to your taste preferences and dietary requirements.

### *Additional Resources and References:*

To learn more about hyperthyroidism and the benefits of smoothies for thyroid health, consider exploring the following resources:

### *Hyperthyroidism Resources:*

American Thyroid Association Provides comprehensive information about thyroid disorders, including hyperthyroidism, its causes, symptoms, and treatment options.

National Institute of Diabetes and Digestive and Kidney Diseases (NIDDK) Offers educational materials on thyroid diseases and their management.

# Testimonials and Reviews:

## Testimonial:

"I cannot express enough how much smoothies have transformed my life with hyperthyroidism. Before, I felt like I had no control over my health. Now, I start my day with a nutrient-packed smoothie that not only nourishes my thyroid but also gives me the energy to take on the world. Thank you for showing me the path to wellness!" - Sarah T.

## Reviews:

"I was skeptical at first, but after trying the smoothie recipes recommended in this guide, I noticed a significant improvement in my energy levels and overall well-being. It's become a daily ritual that I look forward to." - Mark J.

"As someone who has struggled with hyperthyroidism for years, I was searching for natural ways to manage my condition. This comprehensive guide not only explained the benefits of smoothies but also provided delicious recipes that have truly made a difference in my life." - Lisa S.

"The personal story of overcoming hyperthyroidism with smoothies was so inspiring. It gave me hope that I could take control of my health too. I've been making smoothies a regular part of my diet, and I've seen positive changes in my symptoms." - Emma W.

# Chapter: 2

## *60 Hyperthyroidism-Friendly Recipes*

### *1. Green Thyroid Boost Smoothie*

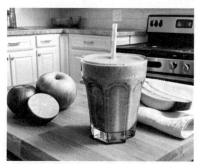

***Description:*** This smoothie is packed with thyroid-supporting ingredients like spinach, kale, and Brazil nuts, providing essential nutrients to help manage hyperthyroidism.

### *Ingredients:*
- 1 cup fresh spinach
- 1/2 cup kale leaves, stems removed
- 1/4 cup Brazil nuts
- 1 ripe banana
- 1 cup unsweetened almond milk
- 1 tablespoon honey (optional)

Ice cubes (optional)

## *Nutritional Information:*

- Calories: 320 kcal
- Protein: 7g
- Carbohydrates: 29g
- Dietary Fiber: 6g
- Fat: 21g
- Sugars: 12g

## *Preparation:*

1. Add spinach, kale, Brazil nuts, banana, and almond milk to a blender.
2. Blend until smooth.
3. Add honey and ice cubes if desired.
4. Blend again until well combined.
5. Pour into a glass and enjoy!

## 2. Blueberry Bliss Thyroid Tonic Smoothie

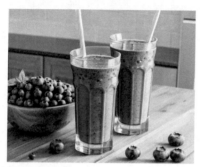

*Description:* This antioxidant-rich smoothie combines blueberries and chia seeds to support thyroid health while providing a burst of delicious flavor.

## Ingredients:

- 1 cup frozen blueberries
- 1 tablespoon chia seeds
- 1/2 cup Greek yogurt
- 1/2 cup unsweetened coconut water
- 1 teaspoon honey (optional)

## Nutritional Information:

- Calories: 220 kcal

- Protein: 10g
  Carbohydrates: 30g
- Dietary Fiber: 7g
- Fat: 7g
- Sugars: 16g

## *Preparation:*

1. Combine frozen blueberries, chia seeds, Greek yogurt, and coconut water in a blender.
2. Blend until smooth and creamy.
3. Add honey if desired for sweetness.
4. Blend briefly to combine.
5. Pour into a glass and serve chilled.

# 3. Mango Madness Thyroid Elixir Smoothie

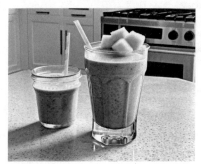

***Description:*** This tropical delight combines mango and coconut for a refreshing smoothie that supports thyroid function and tastes like paradise.

## Ingredients:

- 1 cup fresh mango chunks
- 1/2 cup unsweetened coconut milk
- 1/4 cup plain kefir
- 1 tablespoon shredded coconut (unsweetened)
- 1/2 teaspoon turmeric powder
- 1 teaspoon maple syrup (optional)

## Nutritional Information:

Calories: 270 kcal
Protein: 3g
Carbohydrates: 39g
Dietary Fiber: 5g
Fat: 11g
Sugars: 30g

## Preparation:

1. Place mango chunks, coconut milk, kefir, shredded coconut, and turmeric powder in a blender.
2. Blend until smooth and creamy.
3. Taste and add maple syrup if you desire extra sweetness.
4. Blend briefly to combine.
5. Pour into a glass, garnish with additional shredded coconut if desired, and serve

## 4. Berry Bliss Thyroid Booster Smoothie

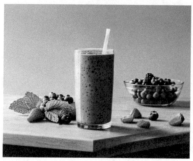

*Description:* A berry-filled smoothie rich in antioxidants, fiber, and essential nutrients to support thyroid health.

## Ingredients:

- 1/2 cup mixed berries (strawberries, blueberries, raspberries)
- 1/2 ripe avocado
- 1/2 cup spinach leaves
- 1/2 cup unsweetened almond milk
- 1 tablespoon flax seeds
- 1 teaspoon honey (optional)

## Nutritional Information:

- Calories: 280 kcal
- Protein: 6g
- Carbohydrates: 24g
- Dietary Fiber: 10g
- Fat: 19g
- Sugars: 9g

## *Preparation:*

1. Combine mixed berries, avocado, spinach, almond milk, and flaxseeds in a blender.
2. Blend until smooth and creamy.
3. Add honey if desired for sweetness.
4. Blend briefly to combine.
5. Pour into a glass and enjoy!

## 5. Nutty Banana Thyroid Tamer Smoothie

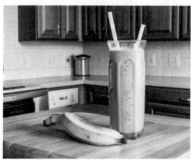

***Description:*** This smoothie is a rich source of selenium and healthy fats from Brazil nuts and almond butter, offering crucial support for your thyroid.

## *Ingredients:*

- 2 ripe bananas
- 1/4 cup Brazil nuts
- 1 tablespoon almond butter
- 1/2 cup unsweetened almond milk
- 1/2 teaspoon cinnamon
- Ice cubes (optional)

## *Nutritional Information:*

- Calories: 340 kcal
- Protein: 7g
- Carbohydrates: 37g
- Dietary Fiber: 7g
- Fat: 20g
- Sugars: 17g

## *Preparation:*

1. Place bananas, Brazil nuts, almond butter, almond milk, and cinnamon in a blender.
2. Blend until smooth.
3. Add ice cubes if you prefer a colder texture.
4. Blend briefly to combine.
5. Pour into a glass and savor the nutty goodness!

# 6. Pineapple Paradise Thyroid Soother Smoothie

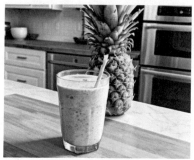

***Description:*** This tropical-inspired smoothie combines pineapple and ginger to soothe inflammation and support thyroid health.

## Ingredients:
- 1 cup fresh pineapple chunks
- 1/2-inch piece of fresh ginger, peeled
- 1/2 cup plain Greek yogurt
- 1/2 cup coconut water
- 1 teaspoon honey (optional)

## Nutritional Information:
- Calories: 190 kcal
- Protein: 7g

- Carbohydrates: 36g
- Dietary Fiber: 3g
- Fat: 2g
- Sugars: 27g

## *Preparation:*

1. Place pineapple chunks, peeled ginger, Greek yogurt, and coconut water in a blender.
2. Blend until smooth and creamy.
3. Add honey if desired for sweetness.
4. Blend briefly to combine.
5. Pour into a glass, garnish with a pineapple slice, and enjoy the tropical goodness!

## 7. Coconut-Berry Thyroid Bliss Smoothie

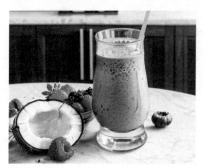

***Description:*** A creamy blend of berries and coconut milk for a delicious and thyroid-supporting smoothie.

## *Ingredients:*

- 1/2 cup mixed berries (strawberries, blueberries, raspberries)
- 1/2 cup unsweetened coconut milk
- 1/4 cup shredded coconut (unsweetened)
- 1/2 teaspoon vanilla extract
- 1 teaspoon honey (optional)

## *Nutritional Information:*

- Calories: 240 kcal
- Protein: 2g
- Carbohydrates: 20g

- Dietary Fiber: 7g
- Fat: 19g
- Sugars: 10g

## *Preparation:*

1. Combine mixed berries, coconut milk, shredded coconut, vanilla extract, and honey (if desired) in a blender.
2. Blend until smooth and creamy.
3. Pour into a glass and sprinkle extra shredded coconut on top for added texture.
4. Sip and enjoy the tropical delight!

# 8. Cinnamon-Apple Thyroid Booster Smoothie

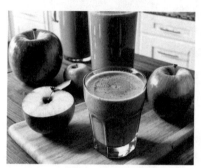

***Description:*** A warm and comforting smoothie that incorporates apples, cinnamon, and oats to support thyroid function.

## *Ingredients:*

- 1 medium apple, peeled and chopped
- 1/4 cup rolled oats
- 1/2 teaspoon ground cinnamon
- 1/2 cup unsweetened almond milk
- 1/2 cup plain Greek yogurt
- 1 teaspoon honey (optional)

## *Nutritional Information:*

- Calories: 280 kcal

- Protein: 7g
- Carbohydrates: 50g
- Dietary Fiber: 9g
- Fat: 6g
- Sugars: 24g

## *Preparation:*

1. Place chopped apple, rolled oats, ground cinnamon, almond milk, Greek yogurt, and honey (if desired) in a blender.
2. Blend until smooth and creamy.
3. Pour into a glass, sprinkle a pinch of cinnamon on top, and savor the cozy flavors.

## 9. Spinach-Mango Thyroid Refresher Smoothie

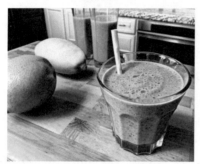

***Description:*** A green smoothie packed with spinach and mango to support thyroid health while providing a refreshing taste.

## Ingredients:

- 1 cup fresh spinach
- 1/2 cup fresh mango chunks
- 1/4 cup plain kefir
- 1/2 cup unsweetened almond milk
- 1 tablespoon chia seeds
- 1 teaspoon honey (optional)

## Nutritional Information:

- Calories: 230 kcal
- Protein: 7g

- Carbohydrates: 34g
- Dietary Fiber: 8g
- Fat: 8g
- Sugars: 22g

## *Preparation:*

1. Add fresh spinach, mango chunks, kefir, almond milk, chia seeds, and honey (if desired) to a blender.
2. Blend until smooth and vibrant green.
3. Pour into a glass, garnish with additional mango slices, and enjoy the refreshing taste.

# 10. Berry-Almond Thyroid Elixir Smoothie

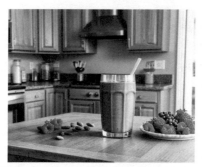

**Description:** A protein-packed smoothie with berries and almond butter to support thyroid function and satisfy your taste buds.

## Ingredients:

- 1/2 cup mixed berries (strawberries, blueberries, raspberries)
- 2 tablespoons almond butter
- 1/2 cup plain Greek yogurt
- 1/2 cup unsweetened almond milk
- 1 tablespoon flax seeds
- 1 teaspoon honey (optional)

## Nutritional Information:

- Calories: 330 kcal
- Protein: 13g
- Carbohydrates: 26g
- Dietary Fiber: 8g
- Fat: 20g
- Sugars: 14g

## *Preparation:*

1. Combine mixed berries, almond butter, Greek yogurt, almond milk, flaxseeds, and honey (if desired) in a blender.
2. Blend until smooth and creamy.
3. Pour into a glass and enjoy the protein-packed goodness

## 11. Papaya Passion Thyroid Support Smoothie

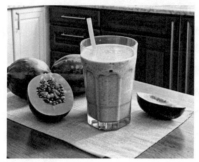

***Description:*** This tropical delight combines papaya, banana, and coconut milk for a soothing and thyroid-supportive smoothie.

## *Ingredients:*

- 1 cup fresh papaya chunks
- 1 ripe banana
- 1/2 cup unsweetened coconut milk
- 1/4 cup Greek yogurt
- 1 tablespoon honey (optional)

## *Nutritional Information:*

- Calories: 270 kcal
- Protein: 4g
- Carbohydrates: 60g
- Dietary Fiber: 5g
- Fat: 5g

- Sugars: 35g

## *Preparation:*

1. Place papaya chunks, ripe banana, coconut milk, Greek yogurt, and honey (if desired) in a blender.
2. Blend until smooth and creamy.
3. Pour into a glass, garnish with a papaya slice, and enjoy the tropical refreshment!

## 12. Cherry-Almond Thyroid Booster Smoothie

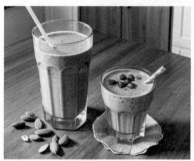

***Description:*** A delightful blend of cherries and almond milk to support thyroid health while satisfying your taste buds.

## *Ingredients:*

- 1 cup frozen cherries
- 1/4 cup unsweetened almond milk
- 1/4 cup plain Greek yogurt
- 2 tablespoons almond butter
- 1/2 teaspoon vanilla extract
- 1 teaspoon honey (optional)

## *Nutritional Information:*

- Calories: 280 kcal

- Protein: 7g
- Carbohydrates: 35g
- Dietary Fiber: 5g
- Fat: 14g
- Sugars: 24g

## *Preparation:*

1. Combine frozen cherries, almond milk, Greek yogurt, almond butter, vanilla extract, and honey (if desired) in a blender.
2. Blend until smooth and creamy.
3. Pour into a glass, garnish with a few extra cherries, and enjoy the delightful flavor.

# 13. Carrot-Cashew Thyroid Elixir Smoothie

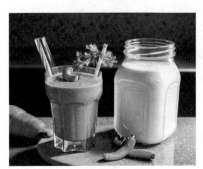

***Description:*** A nutty and nourishing smoothie that incorporates carrots, cashews, and honey for thyroid support.

## Ingredients:

- 1 large carrot, peeled and chopped
- 1/4 cup cashews
- 1/2 cup plain kefir
- 1/2 cup unsweetened almond milk
- 1 tablespoon honey
- 1/2 teaspoon ground cinnamon

## Nutritional Information

- Calories: 290 kcal

- Protein: 8g
- Carbohydrates: 32g
- Dietary Fiber: 5g
- Fat: 16g
- Sugars: 21g

## *Preparation:*

1. Place chopped carrot, cashews, kefir, almond milk, honey, and ground cinnamon in a blender.
2. Blend until smooth and creamy.
3. Pour into a glass, sprinkle a pinch of cinnamon on top, and savor the nutty goodness.

### *14. Mango-Coconut Thyroid Refresher Smoothie*

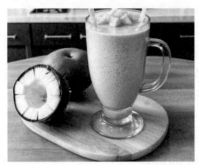

***Description:*** A tropical green smoothie that combines mango, coconut, and spinach for thyroid health and a refreshing taste.

## *Ingredients:*

- 1 cup fresh mango chunks
- 1/2 cup unsweetened coconut milk
- 1/2 cup fresh spinach leaves
- 1 tablespoon shredded coconut (unsweetened)
- 1/2 teaspoon turmeric powder
- 1 teaspoon honey (optional)

## *Nutritional Information:*

- Calories: 250 kcal

- Protein: 3g
- Carbohydrates: 30g
- Dietary Fiber: 5g
- Fat: 12g
- Sugars: 24g

## *Preparation:*

1. Add mango chunks, coconut milk, fresh spinach, shredded coconut, turmeric powder, and honey (if desired) to a blender.
2. Blend until smooth and vibrant green.
3. Pour into a glass, garnish with extra shredded coconut, and enjoy the tropical refreshment.

## 15. Banana-Date Thyroid Tonic Smoothie

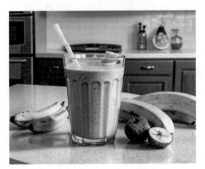

*Description:* A creamy smoothie with banana and dates to provide essential nutrients and support thyroid function.

### Ingredients:

- 2 ripe bananas
- 4-5 pitted dates
- 1/2 cup plain Greek yogurt
- 1/2 cup unsweetened almond milk
- 1/4 teaspoon ground cardamom
- 1 teaspoon honey (optional)

### Nutritional Information:

- Calories: 330 kcal

- Protein: 8g
- Carbohydrates: 70g
- Dietary Fiber: 9g
- Fat: 4g
- Sugars: 45g

## *Preparation:*

1. Combine ripe bananas, pitted dates, Greek yogurt, almond milk, ground cardamom, and honey (if desired) in a blender.
2. Blend until smooth and creamy.
3. Pour into a glass and savor the natural sweetness and creaminess.

# 16. Strawberry-Spinach Thyroid Revive Smoothie

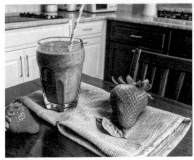

***Description:*** This vibrant green smoothie combines strawberries, spinach, and flaxseeds to provide essential nutrients for thyroid health.

## Ingredients:

- 1 cup fresh strawberries
- 1 cup fresh spinach leaves
- 1 tablespoon flax seeds
- 1/2 cup plain Greek yogurt
- 1/2 cup unsweetened almond milk
- 1 teaspoon honey (optional)

## Nutritional Information:

- Calories: 220 kcal
- Protein: 9g
- Carbohydrates: 33g
- Dietary Fiber: 7g

- Fat: 7g
- Sugars: 20g

## *Preparation:*

1. Place fresh strawberries, spinach leaves, flaxseeds, Greek yogurt, almond milk, and honey (if desired) in a blender.
2. Blend until smooth and vibrant green.
3. Pour into a glass and enjoy the nutrient-packed goodness!

## 17. Blueberry-Banana Thyroid Booster Smoothie

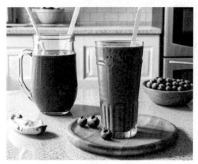

***Description:*** A delightful blend of blueberries, bananas, and almond milk to support thyroid health while providing a burst of delicious flavor.

## Ingredients:

- 1 cup frozen blueberries
- 1 ripe banana
- 1/2 cup unsweetened almond milk
- 1/4 cup plain Greek yogurt
- 1 tablespoon almond butter
- 1 teaspoon honey (optional)

## Nutritional Information:

- Calories: 280 kcal

- Protein: 7g
- Carbohydrates: 45g
- Dietary Fiber: 7g
- Fat: 9g
- Sugars: 28g

## *Preparation:*

1. Combine frozen blueberries, ripe bananas, almond milk, Greek yogurt, almond butter, and honey (if desired) in a blender.
2. Blend until smooth and creamy.
3. Pour into a glass, garnish with a few extra blueberries, and enjoy the delightful flavor.

## *18. Pineapple-Coconut Thyroid Soother Smoothie*

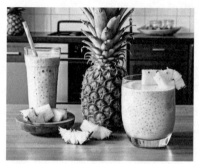

***Description:*** This tropical-inspired smoothie combines pineapple and coconut milk to soothe inflammation and support thyroid health.

## *Ingredients:*

- 1 cup fresh pineapple chunks
- 1/2 cup unsweetened coconut milk
- 1/4 cup plain kefir
- 1/4 cup shredded coconut (unsweetened)
- 1/2 teaspoon ginger powder
- 1 teaspoon honey (optional)

## *Nutritional Information:*

- Calories: 270 kcal

- Protein: 4g
- Carbohydrates: 37g
- Dietary Fiber: 5g
- Fat: 14g
- Sugars: 25g

## *Preparation:*

1. Add fresh pineapple chunks, coconut milk, kefir, shredded coconut, ginger powder, and honey (if desired) to a blender.
2. Blend until smooth and creamy.
3. Pour into a glass, garnish with additional shredded coconut, and enjoy the tropical refreshment.

# 19. Kiwi-Orange Thyroid Tonic Smoothie

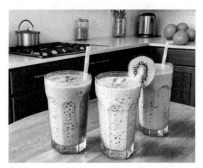

***Description:*** A zesty and vitamin-rich smoothie that incorporates kiwi, orange, and chia seeds to support thyroid function.

## Ingredients:

- 2 ripe kiwis, peeled and chopped
- 1 large orange, peeled and segmented
- 1/2 cup unsweetened orange juice
- 1 tablespoon chia seeds
- 1/2 cup plain Greek yogurt
- 1 teaspoon honey (optional)

## Nutritional Information:

- Calories: 260 kcal

- Protein: 6g
- Carbohydrates: 52g
- Dietary Fiber: 10g
- Fat: 5g
- Sugars: 34g

## *Preparation:*

1. Place chopped kiwis, segmented orange, orange juice, chia seeds, Greek yogurt, and honey (if desired) in a blender.
2. Blend until smooth and zesty.
3. Pour into a glass, garnish with a kiwi slice, and savor the vitamin-rich goodness.

# 20. Raspberry-Beet Thyroid Elixir Smoothie

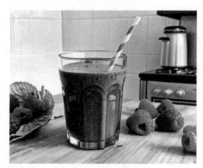

***Description:*** A vibrant red smoothie packed with raspberries, beets, and honey to provide thyroid support and a refreshing taste.

## Ingredients:

- 1 cup frozen raspberries
- 1/2 small beet, peeled and chopped
- 1/2 cup unsweetened almond milk
- 1/2 cup plain Greek yogurt
- 1 tablespoon honey (or more to taste)

## Nutritional Information:

- Calories: 250 kcal
- Protein: 9g

- Carbohydrates: 40g
- Dietary Fiber: 10g
- Fat: 6g
- Sugars: 24g

## *Preparation:*

1. Combine frozen raspberries, chopped beet, almond milk, Greek yogurt, and honey in a blender.
2. Blend until smooth and vibrant red.
3. Pour into a glass, garnish with a fresh raspberry, and enjoy the refreshing taste.

### 21. Lemon-Ginger Thyroid Revitalizer Smoothie

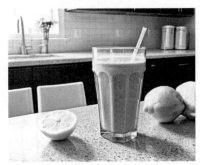

***Description:*** This zesty and invigorating smoothie combines lemon, ginger, and spinach to provide a burst of flavor while supporting thyroid health.

## Ingredients:
- Juice of 1 lemon
- 1/2-inch piece of fresh ginger, peeled
- 1 cup fresh spinach leaves
- 1/2 cup plain Greek yogurt
- 1/2 cup unsweetened almond milk
- 1 teaspoon honey (optional)

## Nutritional Information:
- Calories: 200 kcal
- Protein: 8g
- Carbohydrates: 28g

- Dietary Fiber: 5g
- Fat: 6g
- Sugars: 14g

## *Preparation:*

1. Squeeze the juice of one lemon into a blender.
2. Add the peeled ginger, fresh spinach, Greek yogurt, almond milk, and honey (if desired).
3. Blend until smooth and zesty.
4. Pour into a glass, garnish with a lemon slice, and enjoy the refreshing flavor.

## 22. Avocado-Date Thyroid Booster Smoothie

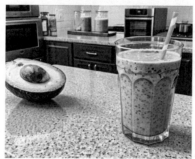

***Description:*** A creamy and nutrient-packed smoothie that combines avocado and dates to support thyroid function and provide a natural sweetness.

## Ingredients:

- 1 ripe avocado
- 4-5 pitted dates
- 1/2 cup unsweetened almond milk
- 1/2 cup plain Greek yogurt
- 1 tablespoon almond butter
- 1 teaspoon honey (optional)

## Nutritional Information:

- Calories: 350 kcal
- Protein: 8g
- Carbohydrates: 47g
- Dietary Fiber: 12g
- Fat: 18g
- Sugars: 30g

## *Preparation:*

1. Scoop out the flesh of the ripe avocado and add it to a blender.
2. Combine with pitted dates, almond milk, Greek yogurt, almond butter, and honey (if desired).
3. Blend until smooth and creamy.
4. Pour into a glass and enjoy the creamy goodness!

## 23. Peach-Cardamom Thyroid Tonic Smoothie

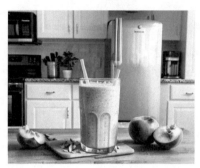

***Description:*** A fragrant and flavorful smoothie that combines peaches and cardamom to support thyroid health and provide a touch of warmth.

## Ingredients:

- 1 cup fresh or frozen peach slices
- 1/2 teaspoon ground cardamom
- 1/2 cup plain Greek yogurt
- 1/2 cup unsweetened almond milk
- 1 tablespoon honey (optional)

## Nutritional Information:

- Calories: 230 kcal
- Protein: 9g

- Carbohydrates: 39g
- Dietary Fiber: 5g
- Fat: 4g
- Sugars: 30g

## *Preparation:*

1. Add fresh or frozen peach slices, ground cardamom, Greek yogurt, almond milk, and honey (if desired) to a blender.
2. Blend until smooth and fragrant.
3. Pour into a glass, sprinkle a pinch of cardamom on top, and savor the aromatic flavor.

## 24. Pomegranate-Walnut Thyroid Elixir Smoothie

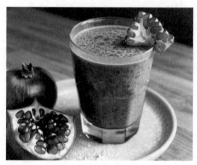

*Description:* A rich and antioxidant-packed smoothie that combines pomegranate and walnuts to support thyroid function and provide a delightful taste.

## Ingredients:

- 1/2 cup pomegranate seeds (from 1 medium pomegranate)
- 1/4 cup walnuts
- 1/2 cup plain kefir
- 1/2 cup unsweetened almond milk
- 1 tablespoon honey (optional)

## Nutritional Information:

- Calories: 280 kcal
- Protein: 8g
- Carbohydrates: 28g
- Dietary Fiber: 4g
- Fat: 16g
- Sugars: 20g

## *Preparation:*

1. Extract the pomegranate seeds from the fruit (or use pre-packaged seeds) and add them to a blender.
2. Combine with walnuts, kefir, almond milk, and honey (if desired).
3. Blend until smooth and rich in color.
4. Pour into a glass, garnish with a few pomegranate seeds, and enjoy the antioxidant goodness!

# 25. Blackberry-Almond Thyroid Booster Smoothie

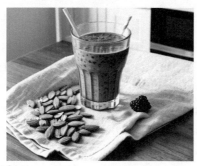

***Description:*** A luscious blend of blackberries and almond milk to support thyroid health while offering a delightful and nutty taste.

## Ingredients:

- 1 cup fresh or frozen blackberries
- 1/2 cup unsweetened almond milk
- 1/4 cup plain Greek yogurt
- 2 tablespoons almond butter
- 1 teaspoon honey (optional)

## Nutritional Information:

- Calories: 240 kcal
- Protein: 7g

- Carbohydrates: 32g
- Dietary Fiber: 10g
- Fat: 11g
- Sugars: 16g

## *Preparation:*

1. Add fresh or frozen blackberries, almond milk, Greek yogurt, almond butter, and honey (if desired) to a blender.
2. Blend until smooth and bursting with blackberry flavor.
3. Pour into a glass, garnish with a few extra blackberries, and enjoy the luscious taste.

# 26. Spinach-Pineapple Thyroid Revive Smoothie

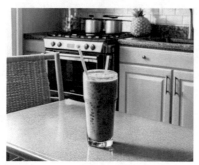

***Description:*** A vibrant green smoothie that combines spinach and pineapple to provide essential nutrients for thyroid health.

## Ingredients:

- 1 cup fresh spinach leaves
- 1 cup fresh pineapple chunks
- 1/2 cup plain Greek yogurt
- 1/2 cup unsweetened coconut water
- 1 teaspoon honey (optional)

## Nutritional Information:

- Calories: 220 kcal
- Protein: 9g
- Carbohydrates: 42g
- Dietary Fiber: 4g
- Fat: 2g
- Sugars: 30g

## Preparation:

1. Place fresh spinach leaves, pineapple chunks, Greek yogurt, coconut water, and honey (if desired) in a blender.
2. Blend until smooth and vibrant green.
3. Pour into a glass, garnish with a pineapple slice, and enjoy the tropical freshness.

## 27. Raspberry-Coconut Thyroid Soother Smoothie

*Description:* A soothing smoothie that combines raspberries and coconut milk to provide a refreshing taste while supporting thyroid health.

## Ingredients:
- 1 cup frozen raspberries
- 1/2 cup unsweetened coconut milk
- 1/4 cup plain Greek yogurt
- 1/4 cup shredded coconut (unsweetened)
- 1 teaspoon honey (optional)

## Nutritional Information:
- Calories: 250 kcal
- Protein: 6g

- Carbohydrates: 35g
- Dietary Fiber: 9g
- Fat: 11g
- Sugars: 18g

## *Preparation:*

1. Combine frozen raspberries, coconut milk, Greek yogurt, shredded coconut, and honey (if desired) in a blender.
2. Blend until smooth and creamy.
3. Pour into a glass, garnish with extra shredded coconut, and enjoy the soothing flavors.

# 28. Mango-Ginger Thyroid Tonic Smoothie

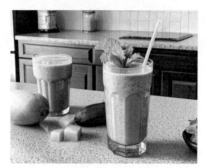

***Description:*** A zingy and tropical smoothie that combines mango and ginger to support thyroid function and provide a refreshing taste.

## *Ingredients:*

- 1 cup fresh mango chunks
- 1/2-inch piece of fresh ginger, peeled
- 1/2 cup plain kefir
- 1/2 cup unsweetened almond milk
- 1 teaspoon honey (optional)

## *Nutritional Information:*

- Calories: 230 kcal
- Protein: 5g

- Carbohydrates: 45g
- Dietary Fiber: 5g
- Fat: 4g
- Sugars: 35g

## *Preparation:*

1. Add fresh mango chunks, peeled ginger, kefir, almond milk, and honey (if desired) to a blender.
2. Blend until smooth and zesty.
3. Pour into a glass, garnish with a mango slice, and enjoy the tropical refreshment.

## 29. Kiwi-Spinach Thyroid Booster Smoothie

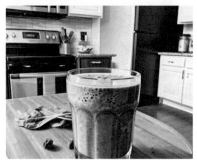

**Description:** A nutrient-packed smoothie that combines kiwi and spinach to support thyroid health while providing a burst of vitamins.

### Ingredients:
- 2 ripe kiwis, peeled and chopped
- 1 cup fresh spinach leaves
- 1/2 cup plain Greek yogurt
- 1/2 cup unsweetened almond milk
- 1 tablespoon honey (optional)

### Nutritional Information:
- Calories: 240 kcal
- Protein: 8g

- Carbohydrates: 42g
- Dietary Fiber: 6g
- Fat: 4g
- Sugars: 27g

## *Preparation:*

1. Place chopped kiwis, fresh spinach leaves, Greek yogurt, almond milk, and honey (if desired) in a blender.
2. Blend until smooth and packed with vitamins.
3. Pour into a glass, garnish with a kiwi slice, and enjoy the nutrient-rich goodness.

## 30. Blueberry-Avocado Thyroid Elixir Smoothie

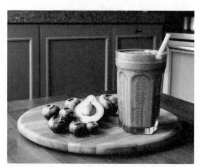

***Description:*** A creamy and antioxidant-rich smoothie that combines blueberries and avocado to support thyroid function and provide a delightful taste.

## Ingredients:

- 1 cup frozen blueberries
- 1/2 ripe avocado
- 1/2 cup unsweetened almond milk
- 1/4 cup plain Greek yogurt
- 1 tablespoon honey (optional)

## Nutritional Information:

- Calories: 280 kcal

- Protein: 7g
- Carbohydrates: 35g
- Dietary Fiber: 10g
- Fat: 14g
- Sugars: 23g

## *Preparation:*

1. Combine frozen blueberries, ripe avocado, almond milk, Greek yogurt, and honey (if desired) in a blender.
2. Blend until smooth and creamy.
3. Pour into a glass, garnish with a few extra blueberries, and enjoy the antioxidant-rich flavor.

## 31. Orange-Mango Thyroid Revive Smoothie

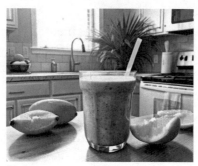

**Description:** A tropical citrus blend of orange and mango to provide essential nutrients for thyroid health and a refreshing taste.

### Ingredients:
- 1 large orange, peeled and segmented
- 1 cup fresh mango chunks
- 1/2 cup plain Greek yogurt
- 1/2 cup unsweetened almond milk
- 1 teaspoon honey (optional)

### Nutritional Information:
- Calories: 220 kcal
- Protein: 9g
- Carbohydrates: 45g
- Dietary Fiber: 7g
- Fat: 3g

- Sugars: 32g

## *Preparation:*

1. Add peeled and segmented orange, fresh mango chunks, Greek yogurt, almond milk, and honey (if desired) to a blender.
2. Blend until smooth and citrusy.
3. Pour into a glass, garnish with an orange slice, and enjoy the tropical refreshment

## 32. Berry-Beet Thyroid Soother Smoothie

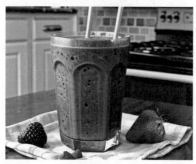

**Description:** A vibrant red smoothie that combines berries and beets to soothe inflammation, support thyroid health, and provide a delightful taste.

### Ingredients:

- 1/2 cup mixed berries (strawberries, blueberries, raspberries)
- 1/2 small beet, peeled and chopped
- 1/2 cup unsweetened almond milk
- 1/4 cup plain Greek yogurt
- 1 tablespoon honey (optional)

### Nutritional Information:

- Calories: 260 kcal
- Protein: 7g
- Carbohydrates: 42g
- Dietary Fiber: 8g
- Fat: 5g
- Sugars: 29g

## *Preparation:*

1. Combine mixed berries, chopped beet, almond milk, Greek yogurt, and honey (if desired) in a blender.
2. Blend until smooth and vibrant red.
3. Pour into a glass, garnish with a few extra berries, and enjoy the antioxidant-rich goodness.

## 33. Spinach-Kiwi Thyroid Tonic Smoothie

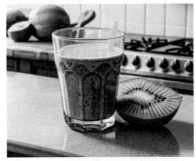

***Description:*** A nutrient-packed green smoothie that combines spinach and kiwi to support thyroid health and provide a burst of vitamins.

## Ingredients:

- 1 cup fresh spinach leaves
- 2 ripe kiwis, peeled and chopped
- 1/2 cup plain Greek yogurt
- 1/2 cup unsweetened almond milk
- 1 teaspoon honey (optional)

## Nutritional Information:

- Calories: 230 kcal
- Protein: 9g

- Carbohydrates: 45g
- Dietary Fiber: 7g
- Fat: 3g
- Sugars: 30g

## *Preparation:*

1. Place fresh spinach leaves, peeled and chopped kiwis, Greek yogurt, almond milk, and honey (if desired) in a blender.
2. Blend until smooth and packed with vitamins.
3. Pour into a glass, garnish with a kiwi slice, and enjoy the nutrient-rich goodness.

## 34. Cherry-Coconut Thyroid Booster Smoothie

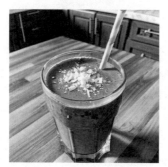

***Description:*** A creamy blend of cherries and coconut milk to support thyroid health while offering a delightful and nutty taste.

## *Ingredients:*

- 1 cup frozen cherries
- 1/2 cup unsweetened coconut milk
- 1/4 cup plain Greek yogurt
- 2 tablespoons almond butter
- 1 teaspoon honey (optional)

## *Nutritional Information:*

- Calories: 270 kcal
- Protein: 7g

- Carbohydrates: 36g
- Dietary Fiber: 5g
- Fat: 13g
- Sugars: 26g

## *Preparation:*

1. Combine frozen cherries, coconut milk, Greek yogurt, almond butter, and honey (if desired) in a blender.
2. Blend until smooth and creamy.
3. Pour into a glass, garnish with a few extra cherries, and enjoy the delightful flavor.

# 35. Banana-Mango Thyroid Elixir Smoothie

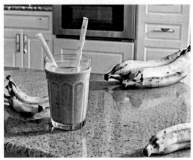

***Description:*** A tropical delight that combines banana and mango to support thyroid function and provide a refreshing taste.

## *Ingredients:*

- 2 ripe bananas
- 1 cup fresh mango chunks
- 1/2 cup plain kefir
- 1/2 cup unsweetened almond milk
- 1 teaspoon honey (optional)

## *Nutritional Information:*

- Calories: 320 kcal
- Protein: 7g

- Carbohydrates: 64g
- Dietary Fiber: 7g
- Fat: 5g
- Sugars: 41g

## *Preparation:*

1. Add ripe bananas, fresh mango chunks, kefir, almond milk, and honey (if desired) to a blender.
2. Blend until smooth and tropical.
3. Pour into a glass, garnish with a mango slice, and enjoy the refreshing taste.

## 36. Almond-Date Thyroid Fuel Smoothie

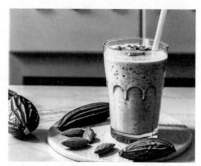

***Description:*** A nourishing blend of almonds and dates to support thyroid health and provide a naturally sweet and nutty flavor.

## *Ingredients:*

- 1/4 cup almonds (soaked and peeled)
- 4-5 pitted dates
- 1/2 cup plain Greek yogurt
- 1/2 cup unsweetened almond milk
- 1 teaspoon honey (optional)

## *Nutritional Information:*

- Calories: 320 kcal
- Protein: 9g
- Carbohydrates: 45g
- Dietary Fiber: 6g
- Fat: 14g
- Sugars: 32g

## Preparation:

1. Soak almonds in water for a few hours, then peel them.
2. Combine soaked and peeled almonds, pitted dates, Greek yogurt, almond milk, and honey (if desired) in a blender.
3. Blend until smooth and creamy.
4. Pour into a glass, garnish with a sprinkle of chopped almonds, and enjoy the nutty goodness!

## 37. Raspberry-Carrot Thyroid Refresher Smoothie

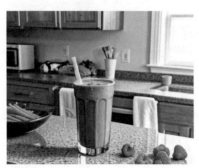

***Description:*** A refreshing blend of raspberries and carrots to support thyroid health while providing a burst of flavor.

## Ingredients:

- 1 cup frozen raspberries
- 1 medium carrot, peeled and chopped
- 1/2 cup plain kefir
- 1/2 cup unsweetened almond milk
- 1 teaspoon honey (optional)

## Nutritional Information:

- Calories: 230 kcal
- Protein: 7g

- Carbohydrates: 40g
- Dietary Fiber: 11g
- Fat: 6g
- Sugars: 25g

## *Preparation:*

1. Combine frozen raspberries, chopped carrot, kefir, almond milk, and honey (if desired) in a blender.
2. Blend until smooth and vibrant red.
3. Pour into a glass, garnish with a raspberry, and enjoy the refreshing taste.

### 38. Spinach-Walnut Thyroid Vitalizer Smoothie

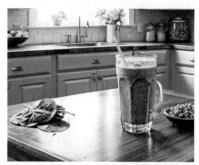

***Description:*** A nutrient-dense green smoothie that combines spinach and walnuts to support thyroid health and provide a rich, nutty flavor.

## Ingredients:
- 1 cup fresh spinach leaves
- 1/4 cup walnuts
- 1/2 cup plain Greek yogurt
- 1/2 cup unsweetened almond milk
- 1 tablespoon honey (optional)

## Nutritional Information:
- Calories: 280 kcal
- Protein: 11g
- Carbohydrates: 24g

- Dietary Fiber: 4g
- Fat: 16g
- Sugars: 16g

## *Preparation:*

1. Place fresh spinach leaves, walnuts, Greek yogurt, almond milk, and honey (if desired) in a blender.
2. Blend until smooth and packed with nutrients.
3. Pour into a glass, garnish with a walnut half, and enjoy the nutty vitality.

### 39. Blueberry-Pomegranate Thyroid Bliss Smoothie

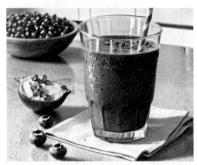

***Description:*** A delightful blend of blueberries and pomegranate to support thyroid health and provide a burst of antioxidant-rich flavor.

### Ingredients:

- 1 cup frozen blueberries
- 1/2 cup pomegranate seeds (from 1 medium pomegranate)
- 1/2 cup plain kefir
- 1/2 cup unsweetened almond milk
- 1 teaspoon honey (optional)

### Nutritional Information:

- Calories: 290 kcal
- Protein: 8g

- Carbohydrates: 42g
- Dietary Fiber: 10g
- Fat: 8g
- Sugars: 28g

## *Preparation:*

1. Combine frozen blueberries, pomegranate seeds, kefir, almond milk, and honey (if desired) in a blender.
2. Blend until smooth and vibrant purple.
3. Pour into a glass, garnish with a sprinkle of additional pomegranate seeds, and enjoy the antioxidant-rich bliss.

## 40. Papaya-Coconut Thyroid Elixir Smoothie

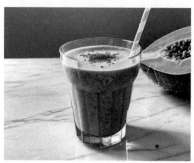

***Description:*** A tropical and creamy smoothie that combines papaya and coconut to soothe inflammation, support thyroid health, and provide a delightful taste.

### Ingredients:

- 1 cup fresh papaya chunks
- 1/2 cup unsweetened coconut milk
- 1/4 cup plain Greek yogurt
- 1/2 teaspoon vanilla extract
- 1 teaspoon honey (optional)

### Nutritional Information:

- Calories: 240 kcal

- Protein: 6g
- Carbohydrates: 42g
- Dietary Fiber: 3g
- Fat: 7g
- Sugars: 32g

## *Preparation:*

1. Add fresh papaya chunks, coconut milk, Greek yogurt, vanilla extract, and honey (if desired) to a blender.
2. Blend until smooth and creamy.
3. Pour into a glass, garnish with a papaya slice, and enjoy the tropical refreshment.

# 41. Apricot-Almond Thyroid Booster Smoothie

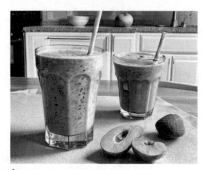

*Description:* A nutty and nutritious smoothie that combines apricots and almonds to support thyroid health and provide a delightful flavor.

## Ingredients:

- 1 cup fresh apricots (pitted)
- 1/4 cup almonds
- 1/2 cup plain Greek yogurt
- 1/2 cup unsweetened almond milk
- 1 teaspoon honey (optional)

## Nutritional Information:

- Calories: 290 kcal
- Protein: 9g
- Carbohydrates: 40g
- Dietary Fiber: 5g

- Fat: 11g
- Sugars: 28g

## *Preparation:*

1. Combine fresh apricots, almonds, Greek yogurt, almond milk, and honey (if desired) in a blender.
2. Blend until smooth and nutty.
3. Pour into a glass, garnish with a sliced apricot, and enjoy the delightful flavor.

## 42. Cherry-Ginger Thyroid Tonic Smoothie

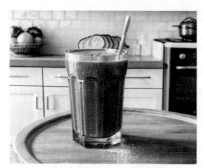

**Description:** A zingy and antioxidant-rich smoothie that combines cherries and ginger to support thyroid function and provide a refreshing taste.

## Ingredients:

- 1 cup frozen cherries
- 1/2-inch piece of fresh ginger, peeled
- 1/2 cup plain kefir
- 1/2 cup unsweetened almond milk
- 1 teaspoon honey (optional)

## Nutritional Information:

- Calories: 240 kcal

- Protein: 6g
- Carbohydrates: 40g
- Dietary Fiber: 4g
- Fat: 7g
- Sugars: 26g

## Preparation:

1. Combine frozen cherries, peeled ginger, kefir, almond milk, and honey (if desired) in a blender.
2. Blend until smooth and zesty.
3. Pour into a glass, garnish with a cherry, and enjoy the antioxidant-rich tonic.

## 43. Pineapple-Basil Thyroid Revive Smoothie

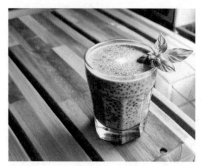

***Description:*** A unique and refreshing smoothie that combines pineapple and basil to support thyroid health and provide a burst of flavor.

## *Ingredients:*

- 1 cup fresh pineapple chunks
- 5-6 fresh basil leaves
- 1/2 cup plain Greek yogurt
- 1/2 cup unsweetened coconut water
- 1 teaspoon honey (optional)

## *Nutritional Information:*

- Calories: 220 kcal
- Protein: 10g
- Carbohydrates: 38g

- Dietary Fiber: 3g
- Fat: 2g
- Sugars: 28g

## *Preparation:*

1. Add fresh pineapple chunks, basil leaves, Greek yogurt, coconut water, and honey (if desired) to a blender.
2. Blend until smooth and aromatic.
3. Pour into a glass, garnish with a basil leaf, and enjoy the unique and refreshing flavor.

### 44. Mango-Cardamom Thyroid Soother Smoothie

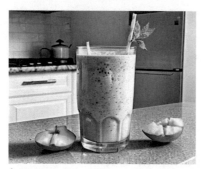

***Description:*** A soothing and fragrant smoothie that combines mango and cardamom to support thyroid health and provide a touch of warmth.

## *Ingredients:*

- 1 cup fresh mango chunks
- 1/2 teaspoon ground cardamom
- 1/2 cup plain Greek yogurt
- 1/2 cup unsweetened almond milk
- 1 teaspoon honey (optional)

## *Nutritional Information:*

- Calories: 230 kcal
- Protein: 7g
- Carbohydrates: 42g

- Dietary Fiber: 4g
- Fat: 4g
- Sugars: 32g

## *Preparation:*

1. Place fresh mango chunks, ground cardamom, Greek yogurt, almond milk, and honey (if desired) in a blender.
2. Blend until smooth and fragrant.
3. Pour into a glass, sprinkle a pinch of cardamom on top, and enjoy the soothing and aromatic taste.

## 45. Blackberry-Pear Thyroid Elixir Smoothie

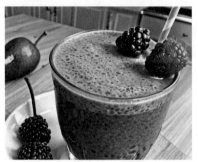

***Description:*** A luscious blend of blackberries and pear to support thyroid health while offering a delightful and juicy flavor.

## Ingredients:

- 1 cup fresh or frozen blackberries
- 1 ripe pear, peeled and chopped
- 1/2 cup plain kefir
- 1/2 cup unsweetened almond milk
- 1 teaspoon honcy (optional)

## Nutritional Information:

- Calories: 260 kcal
- Protein: 7g
- Carbohydrates: 48g
- Dietary Fiber: 11g

- Fat: 6g
- Sugars: 29g

## Preparation:

1. Add fresh or frozen blackberries, chopped pear, kefir, almond milk, and honey (if desired) to a blender.
2. Blend until smooth and bursting with juicy flavor.
3. Pour into a glass, garnish with a blackberry, and enjoy the luscious taste.

## 46. Fig-Walnut Thyroid Vitalizer Smoothie

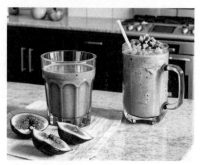

***Description:*** A rich and nutritious smoothie that combines figs and walnuts to support thyroid health and provide a satisfying and nutty flavor.

## Ingredients:

- 1/2 cup dried figs (soaked and chopped)
- 1/4 cup walnuts
- 1/2 cup plain Greek yogurt
- 1/2 cup unsweetened almond milk
- 1 teaspoon honey (optional)

## Nutritional Information:

- Calories: 310 kcal
- Protein: 8g
- Carbohydrates: 45g
- Dietary Fiber: 9g
- Fat: 14g

- Sugars: 33g

## *Preparation:*

1. Soak dried figs in water for a few hours, then chop them.
2. Combine soaked and chopped figs, walnuts, Greek yogurt, almond milk, and honey (if desired) in a blender.
3. Blend until smooth and creamy.
4. Pour into a glass, garnish with a walnut half, and enjoy the nutty vitality.

## 47. Plum-Cardamom Thyroid Tonic Smoothie

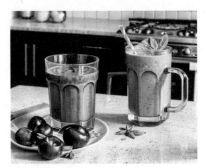

***Description:*** A flavorful and aromatic smoothie that combines plums and cardamom to support thyroid health and provide a unique and soothing taste.

## *Ingredients:*

- 1 cup fresh plum slices (pitted)
- 1/2 teaspoon ground cardamom
- 1/2 cup plain kefir
- 1/2 cup unsweetened almond milk
- 1 teaspoon honey (optional)

## *Nutritional Information:*

- Calories: 240 kcal

- Protein: 7g
- Carbohydrates: 44g
- Dietary Fiber: 7g
- Fat: 4g
- Sugars: 32g

## *Preparation:*

1. Add fresh plum slices, ground cardamom, kefir, almond milk, and honey (if desired) to a blender.
2. Blend until smooth and fragrant.
3. Pour into a glass, sprinkle a pinch of cardamom on top, and enjoy the soothing and aromatic taste.

## 48. Raspberry-Mint Thyroid Refresher Smoothie

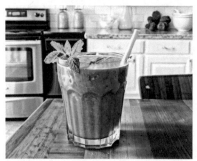

**Description:** A refreshing blend of raspberries and fresh mint leaves to support thyroid health and provide a burst of flavor and cooling sensation.

### Ingredients:

- 1 cup frozen raspberries
- 5-6 fresh mint leaves
- 1/2 cup plain Greek yogurt
- 1/2 cup unsweetened almond milk
- 1 teaspoon honey (optional)

### Nutritional Information:

- Calories: 230 kcal
- Protein: 7g

- Carbohydrates: 40g
- Dietary Fiber: 9g
- Fat: 6g
- Sugars: 25g

## *Preparation:*

1. Combine frozen raspberries, fresh mint leaves, Greek yogurt, almond milk, and honey (if desired) in a blender.
2. Blend until smooth and refreshing.
3. Pour into a glass, garnish with a mint sprig, and enjoy the cooling sensation.

# 49. Guava-Coconut Thyroid Bliss Smoothie

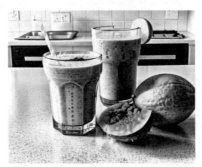

**Description:** A tropical and creamy smoothie that combines guava and coconut to support thyroid health and provide a delightful and exotic flavor.

## Ingredients:
- 1 cup fresh guava chunks (seeds removed)
- 1/2 cup unsweetened coconut milk
- 1/4 cup plain Greek yogurt
- 1/2 teaspoon vanilla extract
- 1 teaspoon honey (optional)

## Nutritional Information:
- Calories: 250 kcal
- Protein: 6g

- Carbohydrates: 40g
- Dietary Fiber: 9g
- Fat: 7g
- Sugars: 29g

## *Preparation:*

1. Add fresh guava chunks (seeds removed), coconut milk, Greek yogurt, vanilla extract, and honey (if desired) to a blender.
2. Blend until smooth and exotic.
3. Pour into a glass, garnish with a guava slice, and enjoy the tropical bliss.

## 50. Kiwi-Basil Thyroid Elixir Smoothie

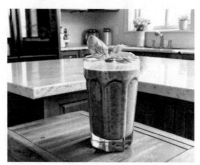

**Description:** A unique and herbaceous smoothie that combines kiwi and basil to support thyroid health and provide a burst of freshness.

## Ingredients:

2 ripe kiwis, peeled and chopped
5-6 fresh basil leaves
1/2 cup plain Greek yogurt
1/2 cup unsweetened almond milk
1 teaspoon honey (optional)

## Nutritional Information:

- Calories: 220 kcal
- Protein: 9g
- Carbohydrates: 45g
- Dietary Fiber: 7g

- Fat: 3g
- Sugars: 30g

## *Preparation:*

1. Place chopped kiwis, fresh basil leaves, Greek yogurt, almond milk, and honey (if desired) in a blender.
2. Blend until smooth and bursting with freshness.
3. Pour into a glass, garnish with a basil leaf, and enjoy the unique and refreshing flavor

### 51. Papaya-Mango Thyroid Revive Smoothie

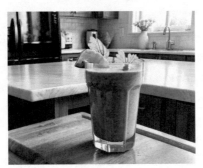

***Description:*** A tropical and vibrant smoothie that combines papaya and mango to support thyroid health and provide a burst of tropical flavor.

## Ingredients:
- 1 cup fresh papaya chunks
- 1 cup fresh mango chunks
- 1/2 cup plain Greek yogurt
- 1/2 cup unsweetened coconut water
- 1 teaspoon honey (optional)

## Nutritional Information:
- Calories: 260 kcal
- Protein: 8g
- Carbohydrates: 53g
- Dietary Fiber: 6g
- Fat: 2g

- Sugars: 38g

## *Preparation:*

1. Add fresh papaya chunks, mango chunks, Greek yogurt, coconut water, and honey (if desired) to a blender.
2. Blend until smooth and bursting with tropical goodness.
3. Pour into a glass, garnish with a slice of papaya or mango, and enjoy the vibrant flavor.

## 52. Blackberry-Lemon Thyroid Booster Smoothie

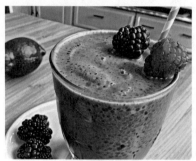

***Description:*** A zesty and antioxidant-rich smoothie that combines blackberries and lemon to support thyroid function and provide a burst of citrus flavor.

### *Ingredients:*

- 1 cup fresh or frozen blackberries
- Juice of 1 lemon
- 1/2 cup plain kefir
- 1/2 cup unsweetened almond milk
- 1 teaspoon honey (optional)

### *Nutritional Information:*

- Calories: 230 kcal

- Protein: 7g
- Carbohydrates: 42g
- Dietary Fiber: 8g
- Fat: 5g
- Sugars: 28g

## *Preparation:*

1. Combine fresh or frozen blackberries, lemon juice, kefir, almond milk, and honey (if desired) in a blender.
2. Blend until smooth and zesty.
3. Pour into a glass, garnish with a lemon twist, and enjoy the citrus burst

## 53. Raspberry-Pineapple Thyroid Elixir Smoothie

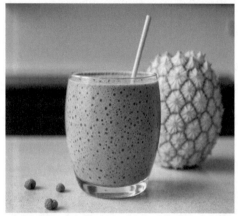

***Description:*** A tropical and antioxidant-packed smoothie that combines raspberries and pineapple to support thyroid health and provide a delightful taste.

## *Ingredients:*

- 1 cup frozen raspberries
- 1 cup fresh pineapple chunks
- 1/2 cup plain Greek yogurt
- 1/2 cup unsweetened coconut water
- 1 teaspoon honey (optional)

## *Nutritional Information:*

- Calories: 240 kcal
- Protein: 9g
- Carbohydrates: 45g
- Dietary Fiber: 9g
- Fat: 2g
- Sugars: 32g

## *Preparation:*

1. Add frozen raspberries, fresh pineapple chunks, Greek yogurt, coconut water, and honey (if desired) to a blender.
2. Blend until smooth and tropical.
3. Pour into a glass, garnish with a pineapple slice, and enjoy the antioxidant-rich elixir.

# 54. Blueberry-Pear Thyroid Tonic Smoothie

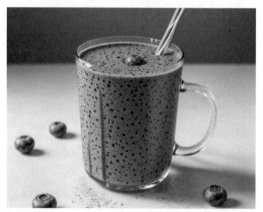

***Description:*** A refreshing and nutrient-packed smoothie that combines blueberries and pear to support thyroid health and provide a delightful taste.

## *Ingredients:*

- 1 cup fresh or frozen blueberries
- 1 ripe pear, peeled and chopped
- 1/2 cup plain kefir
- 1/2 cup unsweetened almond milk
- 1 teaspoon honey (optional)

## *Nutritional Information:*

- Calories: 250 kcal
- Protein: 8g
- Carbohydrates: 48g
- Dietary Fiber: 11g
- Fat: 4g
- Sugars: 31g

## *Preparation:*

1. Combine fresh or frozen blueberries, chopped pear, kefir, almond milk, and honey (if desired) in a blender.
2. Blend until smooth and packed with nutrients.
3. Pour into a glass, garnish with a blueberry or pear slice, and enjoy the refreshing tonic.

## 55. Mango-Passion Fruit Thyroid Bliss Smoothie

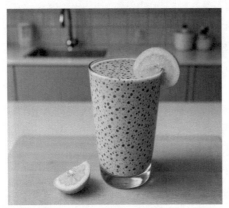

***Description:*** An exotic and creamy smoothie that combines mango and passion fruit to support thyroid health and provide a delightful and tangy flavor.

### Ingredients:

- 1 cup fresh mango chunks
- Pulp of 2 passion fruits
- 1/2 cup plain Greek yogurt
- 1/2 cup unsweetened coconut milk
- 1 teaspoon honey (optional)

### Nutritional Information:

- Calories: 280 kcal

- Protein: 6g
- Carbohydrates: 50g
- Dietary Fiber: 7g
- Fat: 6g
- Sugars: 37g

## *Preparation:*

1. Add fresh mango chunks, pulp of passion fruits, Greek yogurt, coconut milk, and honey (if desired) to a blender.
2. Blend until smooth and exotic.
3. Pour into a glass, garnish with a passion fruit pulp, and enjoy the tropical bliss.

## 56. Kiwi-Strawberry Thyroid Vitalizer Smoothie

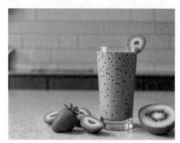

*Description:* A vibrant and vitamin-packed smoothie that combines kiwi and strawberries to support thyroid health and provide a refreshing taste.

## Ingredients:

- 2 ripe kiwis, peeled and chopped
- 1 cup fresh strawberries, hulled
- 1/2 cup plain Greek yogurt
- 1/2 cup unsweetened almond milk
- 1 teaspoon honey (optional)

## Nutritional Information:

- Calories: 240 kcal
- Protein: 8g

- Carbohydrates: 48g
- Dietary Fiber: 9g
- Fat: 4g
- Sugars: 29g

## *Preparation:*

1. Place chopped kiwis, fresh strawberries, Greek yogurt, almond milk, and honey (if desired) in a blender.
2. Blend until smooth and bursting with vitamins.
3. Pour into a glass, garnish with a kiwi slice, and enjoy the nutrient-rich goodness.

## 57. Raspberry-Mint Thyroid Revive Smoothie

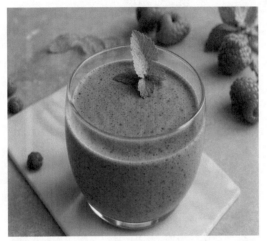

***Description:*** A refreshing and antioxidant-rich smoothie that combines raspberries and fresh mint leaves to support thyroid health and provide a burst of flavor.

### *Ingredients:*
1 cup frozen raspberries
5-6 fresh mint leaves
1/2 cup plain kefir
1/2 cup unsweetened coconut water
1 teaspoon honey (optional)

## Nutritional Information:

- Calories: 220 kcal
- Protein: 7g
- Carbohydrates: 40g
- Dietary Fiber: 9g
- Fat: 5g
- Sugars: 25g

## Preparation:

1. Combine frozen raspberries, fresh mint leaves, kefir, coconut water, and honey (if desired) in a blender.
2. Blend until smooth and refreshing.
3. Pour into a glass, garnish with a mint sprig, and enjoy the cooling sensation.

## 58. Peach-Almond Thyroid Booster Smoothie

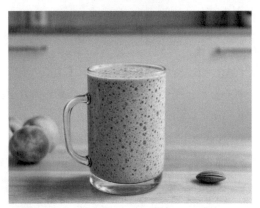

**Description:** A nutty and delicious smoothie that combines peaches and almonds to support thyroid health and provide a delightful flavor.

### Ingredients:
- 1 cup fresh peach slices (peeled)
- 1/4 cup almonds
- 1/2 cup plain Greek yogurt
- 1/2 cup unsweetened almond milk
- 1 teaspoon honey (optional)

### Nutritional Information:
- Calories: 280 kcal

- Protein: 9g
- Carbohydrates: 40g
- Dietary Fiber: 6g
- Fat: 11g
- Sugars: 33g

## *Preparation:*

1. Add fresh peach slices, almonds, Greek yogurt, almond milk, and honey (if desired) to a blender.
2. Blend until smooth and nutty.
3. Pour into a glass, garnish with a peach slice, and enjoy the delightful flavor.

## 59. Blueberry-Coconut Thyroid Elixir Smoothie

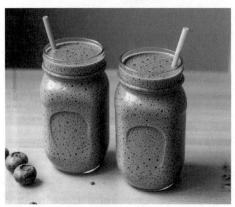

***Description:*** A tropical and antioxidant-rich smoothie that combines blueberries and coconut to support thyroid health and provide a delightful taste.

## *Ingredients:*

- 1 cup frozen blueberries
- 1/2 cup unsweetened coconut milk
- 1/4 cup plain Greek yogurt
- 2 tablespoons shredded coconut (unsweetened)
- 1 teaspoon honey (optional)

## *Nutritional Information:*

- Calories: 270 kcal
- Protein: 7g
- Carbohydrates: 45g
- Dietary Fiber: 10g
- Fat: 8g
- Sugars: 28g

## *Preparation:*

1. Combine frozen blueberries, coconut milk, Greek yogurt, shredded coconut, and honey (if desired) in a blender.
2. Blend until smooth and creamy.
3. Pour into a glass, garnish with a sprinkle of shredded coconut, and enjoy the antioxidant-rich flavor.

## 60. Pineapple-Orange Thyroid Soother Smoothie

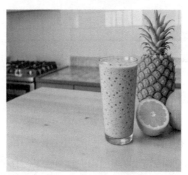

***Description:*** A tropical and citrusy smoothie that combines pineapple and orange to support thyroid health and provide a refreshing taste.

## *Ingredients:*

- 1 cup fresh pineapple chunks
- Juice of 1 orange
- 1/2 cup plain kefir
- 1/2 cup unsweetened coconut water
- 1 teaspoon honey (optional)

## *Nutritional Information:*

- Calories: 230 kcal
- Protein: 6g

- Carbohydrates: 45g
- Dietary Fiber: 3g
- Fat: 2g
- Sugars: 30g

## *Preparation:*

1. Add fresh pineapple chunks, orange juice, kefir, coconut water, and honey (if desired) to a blender.
2. Blend until smooth and citrusy.
3. Pour into a glass, garnish with a pineapple slice, and enjoy the tropical refreshment.

## *Conclusion:*

In closing, *"Hyperthyroidism Smoothies Book"* has taken you on a journey to discover the incredible power of nutrition in managing hyperthyroidism. I have explored the nuances of this thyroid disorder, delved into the world of nourishing smoothies, and provided you with a wide array of delicious recipes designed to support your thyroid health while tantalizing your taste buds.

Remember that managing hyperthyroidism is not just about medical treatments; it's about making everyday choices that promote wellness. Incorporating these smoothies into your daily routine can be a transformative step toward better health. With the right ingredients and knowledge, you have the tools to enhance your well-being and embark on a path to optimal thyroid function.

As you sip your vibrant smoothies, may you find comfort and healing in each delicious sip. Here's to vibrant health, boundless energy, and a life well-lived!

I would like to express my heartfelt gratitude for choosing *"Hyperthyroidism Smoothies Book"* as your trusted companion on your journey to better health. Your decision to explore the power of nutrition in managing hyperthyroidism is a commendable one, and we are honored to have been a part of your wellness journey.

Your support and dedication to your health inspire us every day. I hope that the knowledge and recipes shared in this book have been informative, empowering, and enjoyable for you. Your well-being is my utmost priority, and I believe that with the right tools and understanding, you can take control of your health and thrive despite the challenges of hyperthyroidism.

As you embark on this path of nourishment and healing, remember that small changes can lead to significant improvements in your health. I encourage you to continue exploring the world of nutritious smoothies and making choices that promote vitality and well-being.

Once again, thank you for placing your trust in me.I wish you all the health, happiness, and smoothie-filled days ahead!

**With warm regards,**
**KELLY D.LYONS**
*Author of "Hyperthyroidism Smoothies Book"*

Made in the USA
Columbia, SC
27 June 2024

37812164R00083